# HEART HEALTHY FOOD

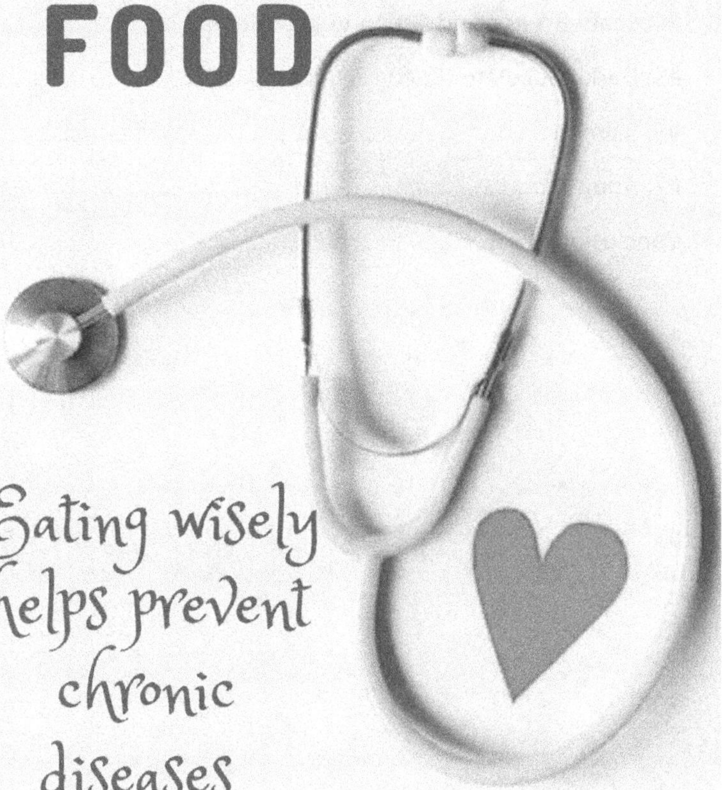

Eating wisely helps prevent chronic diseases

Discover 7 ways to power up, wind down, and have fun.

By Dr. John Adams

# Table of Contents

## Introduction

Do you want to live a healthy, long life? Although we are all aware that we cannot live forever, we may take good care of our health by giving our bodies the best treatment, which will inevitably help us live longer.

According to studies, professionals have shown that people who consistently eat meals that serve to fuel the body for maximum health tend to live longer and healthier lives. In other words, they avoid processed, packaged, or additive-containing foods and only eat items that are healthy for their bodies.

We still have influence over our health and nutritional choices, even though there is a potential that heredity may predispose us to many different diseases. Although there are no certainties regarding how long we will live or how our health will be as we age, there are practical activities that may be taken to have a happier and more fulfilling life. Below we'll talk about 7 meals that are good for your heart and help you live longer.

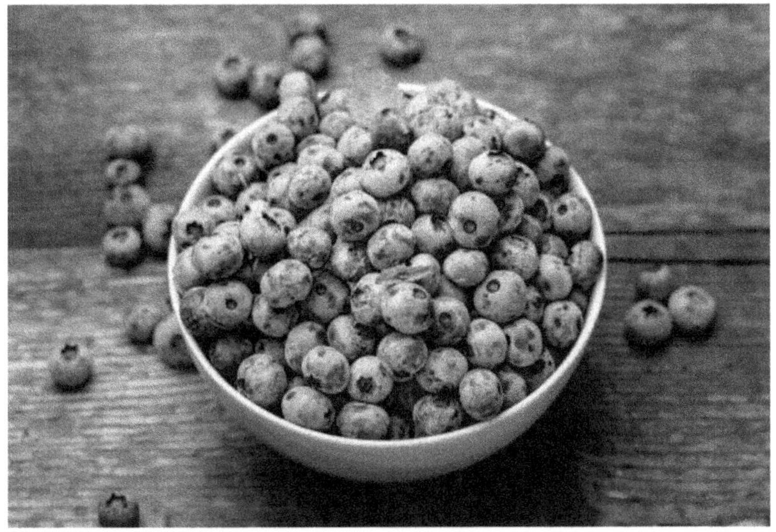

## *#1*: Blueberries

Because they can prevent and even reverse the majority of the effects of aging, blueberries have been dubbed "superfruits." They are amazing anti-aging foods that maintain the health of the brain by enhancing mental health. Berries' dark coloring reveals their high antioxidant content, which fights free radicals that cause aging and prevents the growth of new cells to maintain health.

Blueberries are not only a potent source of antioxidants with numerous health advantages, but they can also slow down certain aging processes. Blueberry extracts have been demonstrated to significantly lengthen life, according to recent studies. Additionally, blueberries have the most nutrients per calorie of any fruit. Also possible with regular ingestion is a decrease in belly fat.

Blueberries make a terrific choice for a quick guilt-free snack because they contain less sugar than other fruits and are therefore less likely to have an impact on your insulin levels. Low-glycemic fruits aid in maintaining a healthy insulin balance as well as mental clarity. These fruits are also rich in fiber, which supports healthy weight development and longevity by keeping digestion on track, maintaining cholesterol levels, and lowering blood pressure.

Berries of all varieties are nutritious because they contain high concentrations of phytochemicals that protect against cancer, DNA damage, metabolic syndrome, and heart disease. Blood vessels will become more flexible as a result, reducing the possibility of getting heart disease. The specific favonoid components of blueberries, rather than the entire fruit, are what provide so many health advantages. These substances can improve high blood pressure, lower cardiovascular risk factors, and help the brain recover quickly from a stroke. Recent research has shown that blueberries protect memory-related brain areas from potential oxidative and inflammatory harm and aid in preventing brain degeneration.

Because they are so rich in pterostilbenes and anthocyanins, blueberries are increasingly important in programs for extending life based on research. Researchers have uncovered new evidence that blueberries can prevent aging and promote longevity.

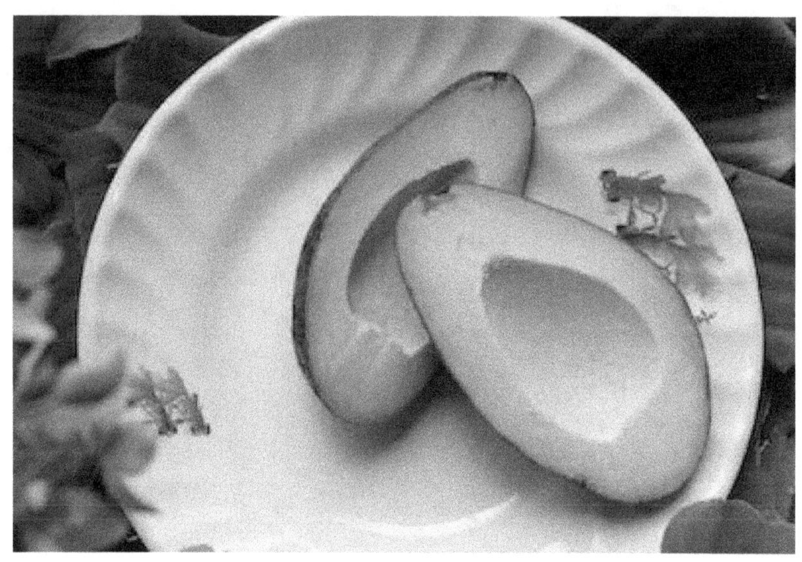

## #2: Avocados

People eat avocados not just for their distinct flavor but also for their outstanding heart health advantages. Avocados are one of the healthiest foods since they are packed with nutrients including folic acid, protein, magnesium, vitamin E, and other B vitamins. Additionally, they are a wonderful source of lipids that reduce inflammation and slow down the body's aging process.

Avocados are abundant in mono- and polyunsaturated fats, which make it simple to produce energy, said a dietician in Washington. As a result, the risk of heart disease and blood cholesterol levels can be reduced. This fruit increases levels of good cholesterol in addition to lowering levels of bad cholesterol. According to Reader's Digest, foods with high monounsaturated fat content can reduce insulin resistance, which helps to control blood sugar levels. Of all the fruits, avocado's low carb and sugar content aids in improved blood sugar regulation. Aside from that, avocados' high potassium content aids in maintaining normal blood pressure.

Compared to processed or animal-based fats, avocados are a more readily digested and absorbed type of fat since they are a water-rich food. Avocados are best consumed when they are ripe because this is when their nutrients have fully formed and are most easily tolerated. In addition to acting as a superb all-purpose food to sate desires, avocado may also be substituted for fat when baking. Additionally, you can use it to replace some of your favorite dairy recipes. In addition, it can be included in other recipes such as soups and dessert whips.

Avocado consumption has been linked to a number of beneficial health consequences, including improved appetite control and weight management, according to research. In 2013, a Nutrition Journal article based on a 7-year review found that avocados are associated with a reduced risk of metabolic syndrome, a condition in which a number of symptoms are present and may raise the risk of diabetes, stroke, and cardiovascular disease. It also makes it possible for the body to absorb other nutrients more effectively.

In addition, studies have shown that avocados can improve cholesterol levels in as little as a week, contain chemicals that inhibit and kill oral cancer cells, and provide protection against liver damage. Despite the fact that eating avocados has many health advantages, overindulging in this fruit can lead to weight gain because of the high fat content. As fat takes longer to absorb than other nutrients, keeping you feeling fuller for longer, it may also As fat takes longer to absorb than other nutrients, keeping you feeling fuller for longer, it may also result in nutritional shortages.

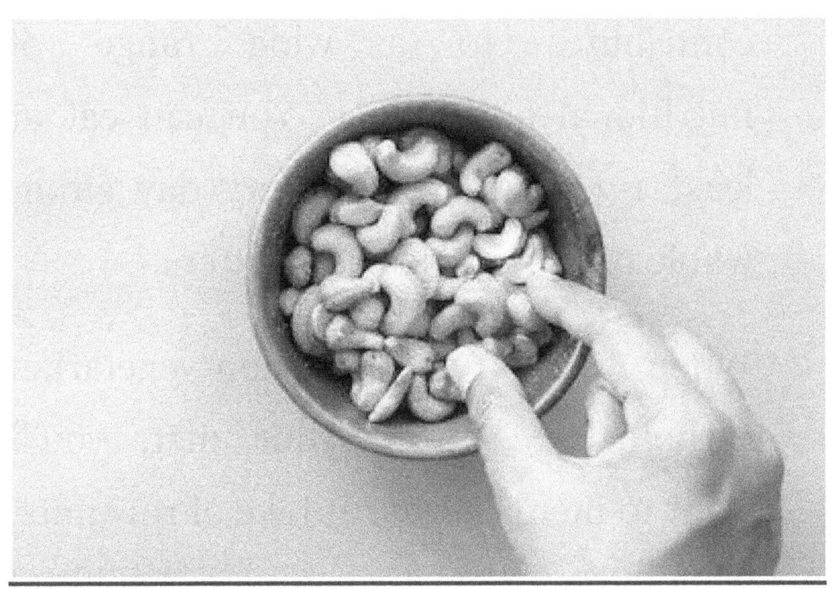

### #3: Walnuts (and other Nuts and Seeds)

It is vitally important for excellent health to add nutrients like nuts and seeds to your longevity diet plan as a supplement. They are an excellent source of the dietary fiber needed to maintain good health. Recent studies have revealed that eating walnuts in their entirety, including the skin, contributes to a wide range of nutritional advantages. You can eat at least 1-3 ounces of it every day either whole or as nut and seed butters.

When you cut out non-vegetarian carbohydrates from your diet, you'll want to increase your intake of raw nuts, which are a fantastic source of healthful fats. They are an excellent snack when energy starts to wane because they are sufficiently fortified with minerals and vitamins. These heart-healthy ingredients can also be included in a variety of recipes to add flavor and additional nutrients. First off, they largely consist of heart-healthy unsaturated fats. They aid in reducing inflammation throughout the body, particularly in the blood and heart.

Omega-3 fatty acids, which are found in walnuts, assist people maintain healthy weight, boost heart health, and ensure that their brains are functioning properly. According to a recent scientific study, children who are deficient in the omega-3 fatty acids found in walnuts might become hyperactive, irritable, and throw tantrums. A child's mood can be lifted and their EFAs shortfall is reduced by including walnuts in their diet. Even grownups who are experiencing stress and sadness can use it. Omega-3 fatty acids can be found in seeds, flax, and hemp seeds, among other foods.

Other nuts, including almonds and cashews, are also rich providers of magnesium and iron, which support a balanced metabolism and prevent weariness and high insulin levels. In addition to having a high fat content, seeds and nuts can assist in regulating metabolism and reducing cravings for harmful meals. But not all nuts are created equal; some may include higher levels of protein, carbohydrates, or healthful fat.

According to a 30-year study, those who ate nuts at least seven times per week at a minimum of one ounce each serving had a 20% higher chance of living longer than those who did not. There will be a general decrease in the chance of death from heart disease, cancer, and respiratory diseases if nuts are consumed at least five times a week.

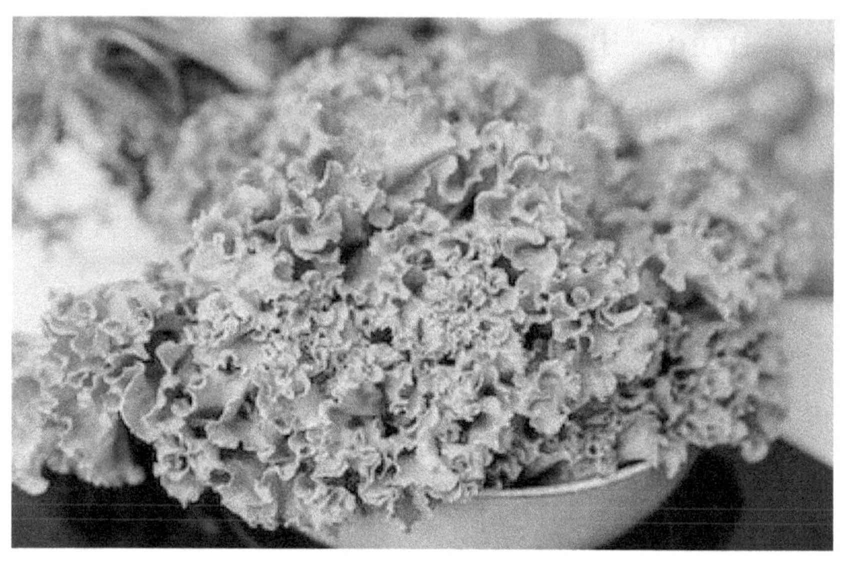

### #4: Leafy Greens and Green Vegetables

Green veggies are good for your heart and are a cornerstone of every balanced diet and lifestyle plan. They are the most alkaline meals that can be found all year long and are stocked with enough vitamins, protein, and minerals. The greatest leafy green vegetables to eat are those that are high in protein, calcium, magnesium, chlorophyll, and iron.

Examples of these veggies include broccoli, kale, and spinach.

Leafy green veggies also include vitamins A and C in addition to vitamin B6. The high vitamin K level of kale helps to develop bones, which is important for year-round activity. Leafy greens are also known to be the best anti-cancer meals, helping to prevent cancer in its early stages and even changing the course of some serious health issues. They are loaded with a lot of carotenoids, antioxidants, and other chemicals made for illness prevention. The antioxidants protect the heart against cardiovascular disease and aid in the prevention of some birth abnormalities.

Additionally, the vitamin in leafy green vegetables decreases homocysteine levels, reducing the risk of heart disease. The fact that dark leafy greens have low levels of calories, carbs, and glycemic index is one of its most alluring advantages. These qualities make it easier for individuals to achieve and maintain a healthy body weight. Increased dietary fiber intake from adding more green vegetables to a balanced diet aids in weight management, intestinal health, and digestive system control.

A gene called T-bet has been shown to respond specifically to leafy greens, according to researchers. These immune cells are essential for the development of immune cells that are found in your gut, which are in charge of treating inflammatory illnesses and may even lower your chance of developing bowel cancer. There are significant health benefits that those who consume three or more servings of dark leafy greens daily are missing out on.

Vegetables are a varied food group, offering a vast selection and enough to satisfy everyone's tastes and preferences. By juicing your vegetables with sprouted beans, you may improve your vegetable consumption in the simplest and most efficient method possible. This is so that your body can absorb every nutrient in the veggies, although some micronutrients may be lost during cooking, juicing makes them easily digestible. According to a featured article, people in their middle years who consume a cup of cooked greens every day tend to live longer than those who don't include leafy greens in their diet.

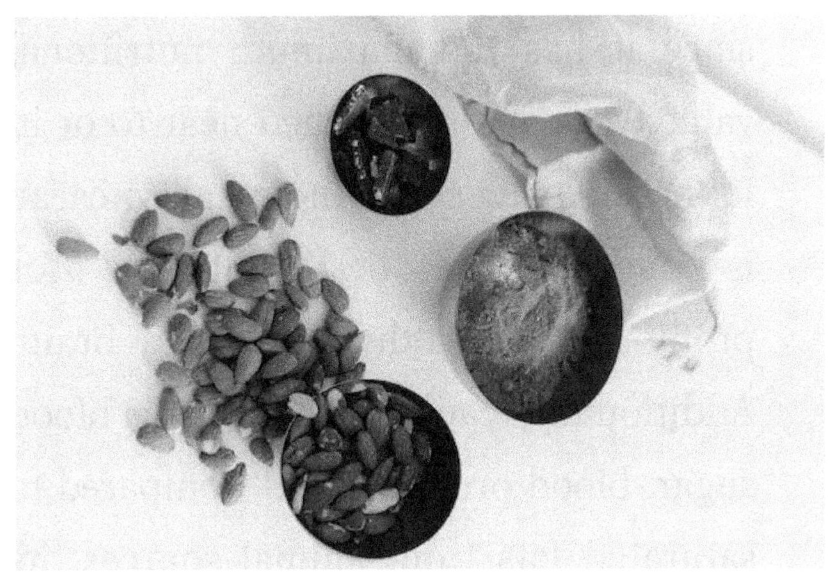

### #5: Dark Chocolate (Cocoa & Cacao)

According to research, eating decadent dark chocolate provides more than 40 different nutritional advantages, including a longer lifespan. Since it is manufactured from cocoa seeds, dark chocolate is one of the world's best sources of antioxidants. It works best when cacao (cocoa) is consumed raw since it has the maximum nutritional value when it is consumed near to or in its natural raw state. In actuality, cacao is one of the best nutrients for promoting a healthy heart and brain. Additionally, cacao helps reduce blood sugar, blood pressure, and Compared to saturated fats from animal sources, its healthy fats are really good for your body.

According to a 2007 study published in the Journal of Nutrition, dark chocolate contains a lot of flavonoids, an antioxidant class that has been shown to prevent cardiovascular disease. Furthermore, eating high-cocoa-content, high-quality dark chocolate is better for you, especially if it has at least 70% cocoa. Both raw cacao and cocoa are fantastic heart-healthy foods that improve hormone production, blood flow, and even digestion.

Basically, due to the numerous health advantages it provides, dark chocolate may be the greatest option if you want to treat yourself to a sweet snack while also maintaining your health. But keep in mind that it also contains a lot of fat. You might choose organic cocoa powder or raw cacao powder in addition to monitoring your fat intake. Consuming dark chocolate regularly aids in the breakdown of bacteria and the fermentation of its ingredients into anti-inflammatory substances, both of which are ultimately beneficial to your long-term health. In addition, dark chocolate promotes healthy blood circulation and reduces the risk of blood clots.

Due to the presence of several chemical constituents that have a good impact on your mind, dark chocolate also serves as a mood enhancer. It contains phenylethylamine (PEA), which enables the release of endorphins in the brain. Consuming dark chocolate will therefore assist to lift your spirits and make you happier. According to a 1999 Harvard study of 8000 males, those who consumed dark chocolate at least three times each month were able to live an additional year than those who did not.

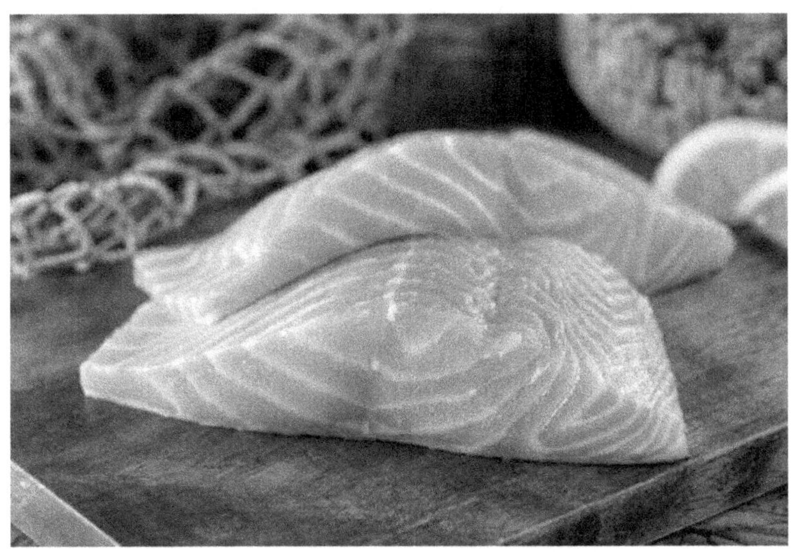

### #6: Salmon

Salmon is not only delicious, but it also has a number of positive health benefits. Salmon is a nutritional powerhouse that is rich in vitamin D and omega-3 fatty acids. It has been demonstrated that omega-3s can reduce triglyceride levels and the risk of inflammation, both of which are associated with an increased risk of heart disease. There is proof that omega-3 fatty acids maintain the brain healthy by reducing the risk of dementia and cognitive decline.

Additionally, giving preschoolers salmon reduces their likelihood of developing ADHD symptoms and can improve their academic performance because salmon's nutrients helps kids concentrate and remember things better. According to studies, salmon's omega-3 fatty acids may encourage weight loss and considerably reduce abdominal fat in obese people. Salmon is a particularly nutritous nutritional choice because it only has a minimum amount of the potentially dangerous pollutant mercury, while the majority of fatty fish are filled with omega-3s.

Other health advantages of salmon may have been forgotten in the focus on the omega-3 benefits. Salmon's protein and amino acid content are connected to yet another advantage. Researchers have found that salmon contains tiny bioactive protein molecules known as bioactive peptides that can cure joint cartilage, reduce insulin resistance, and manage gastrointestinal inflammation.

Additionally, salmon has a high potassium content, which can lower blood pressure and stop fatty deposits from accumulating in the arteries. According to a new study, eating salmon with the bones is more advantageous since it is a wonderful source of calcium, which helps to maintain the health of your bones. Regular salmon consumption lowers the risk of cognitive decline in older people as well as depression and aggression in adolescents. Salmon consumption throughout pregnancy aids in maintaining the fetal brain's health and protection.

Salmon may be prepared in a variety of creative ways in the kitchen, making it incredibly flexible. However, purchasing salmon in cans is a simple and affordable substitute that provides the same health benefits as eating fresh fish. Simply said, including at least two servings of this fatty fish in your normal diet will help you satisfy your nutrient demands and reduce your chance of contracting certain ailments.

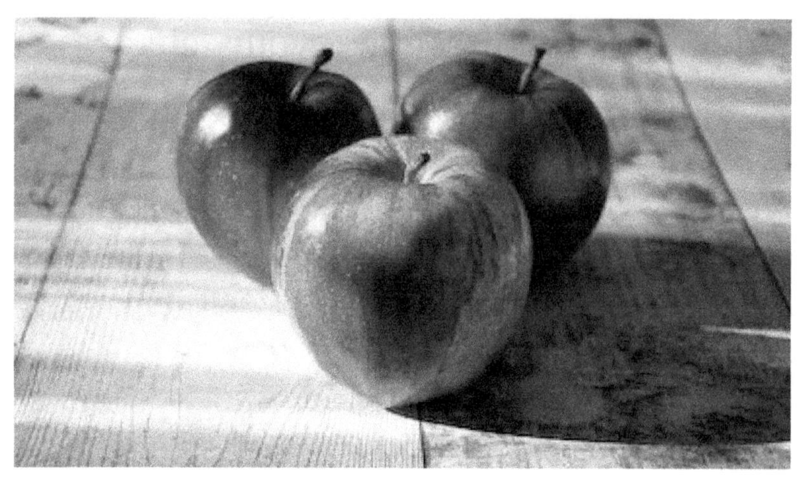

#### #7: Apple

Several studies suggest that including apples in your longevity diet may make them one of the healthiest fruits in the world. Despite being the most consumed fruit, individuals frequently ignore their remarkable health advantages. In fact, apples were ranked #1 among the other foods in a Medical News Today feature article on the top 10. An apple a day may be the best food to prolong lifespan because it has so many health benefits, proving the old adage that we are all familiar with.

First off, apples are a good source of vitamin C, fiber, a number of antioxidants, and folate, which can help prevent Alzheimer's. Additionally, they have oxidants called polyphenols, which are predominantly concentrated in the peel and serve this purpose. Therefore, it is better to eat the apple's peel in order to reap the most benefits. These polyphenols contain quercetin, a flavonoid that lowers blood pressure. According to studies, eating a lot of flavonoids has been linked to a 20% lower risk of stroke. It was determined by researchers that eating apples high in flavonoids could reduce the risk of developing pancreatic cancer by 23%.

By citing Flores, it was mentioned that frequent apple consumption has been shown to have positive effects on the heart because of the high fiber and polyphenol content of apples. The antioxidant content of apples ranks best among all other fruits when it comes to lowering the chance of acquiring cancer, particularly lung cancer, according to Flores. Another study compares the effects of eating an apple a day to statins, a class of medications used to decrease cholesterol levels. According to estimates, apples are virtually as beneficial as statins at reducing mortality.

In a nutshell, apples are a fantastic food choice for promoting lifespan and good health because they include a number of elements that set them apart from other fruits.

## Conclusion

Making wise food decisions is crucial in determining how our lives will change over time. While there is no one food that can cure all ailments, eating a variety of healthful foods regularly can help you stay disease-free and improve your general health. Long-term benefits of including such heart-healthy items in your diet are unquestionably possible. An completely better life, longer life, and better health are just a decision away!

www.ingramcontent.com/pod-product-compliance
Lightning Source LLC
LaVergne TN
LVHW020534160826
845677LV00015B/4050

* 9 7 9 8 3 6 8 2 1 9 5 7 8 *